BLOOD SUGAR DIET SOLUTION FOR SENIORS

A Comprehensive Guide to Managing Diabetes with Healthy, Low-Carbs Recipes.

By

Hector Wiggins

Table of Contents

INTRODUCTION

In the quiet town of Elderview, where the streets echoed with the tales of a life well-lived, a whisper began to circulate among the community's seniors. It was a whisper that spoke of vitality, renewed energy, and a pathway to gracefully navigate the golden years with a bounce in their step. At the heart of this hushed conversation was a groundbreaking guide, a beacon of health for Elderview's seniors – the "Blood Sugar Diet Solution for Seniors."

The story unfolded as Dr. Margaret Turner, a seasoned geriatrician with a heart dedicated to the well-being of her community, observed a common thread weaving through the lives of her elderly patients. The challenge of managing blood sugar levels was an intricate dance that impacted not only their physical health but also their zest for life.

Determined to script a new narrative for Elderview's seniors, Dr. Turner delved into the intricate connection between aging and blood sugar regulation. Her quest for a solution led to a compilation of wisdom, science, and practical strategies tailored specifically for the unique needs of the town's cherished older residents.

The book, "Blood Sugar Diet Solution for Seniors," became a testament to Dr. Turner's commitment to empowering the elderly with knowledge and actionable steps. It wasn't just a guide; it was a roadmap to a vibrant, healthy, and fulfilling chapter of life.

As the pages turned, Elderview's seniors discovered the secrets of crafting nutritious meals that nourished both body and soul. They embarked on gentle yet effective exercise routines, discovering the joy of movement that defied the stereotypes of aging.

The aroma of wholesome recipes wafted through the air, filling kitchens with the promise of a balanced and delectable diet.

In this narrative, community members found more than just a health manual – they found a companion for their journey. The book's guidance wasn't merely about blood sugar; it was about reclaiming a sense of control, fostering resilience, and embracing a life rich in experiences.

And so, in Elderview, a transformation began. Seniors embraced the "Blood Sugar Diet Solution" not as a prescription but as a passport to a future where age was just a number, and the best chapters were yet to be written. Dr. Turner's creation became a source of inspiration, a bridge connecting generations, and a legacy that would resonate through the years, echoing the importance of health, vitality, and the joy of living well.

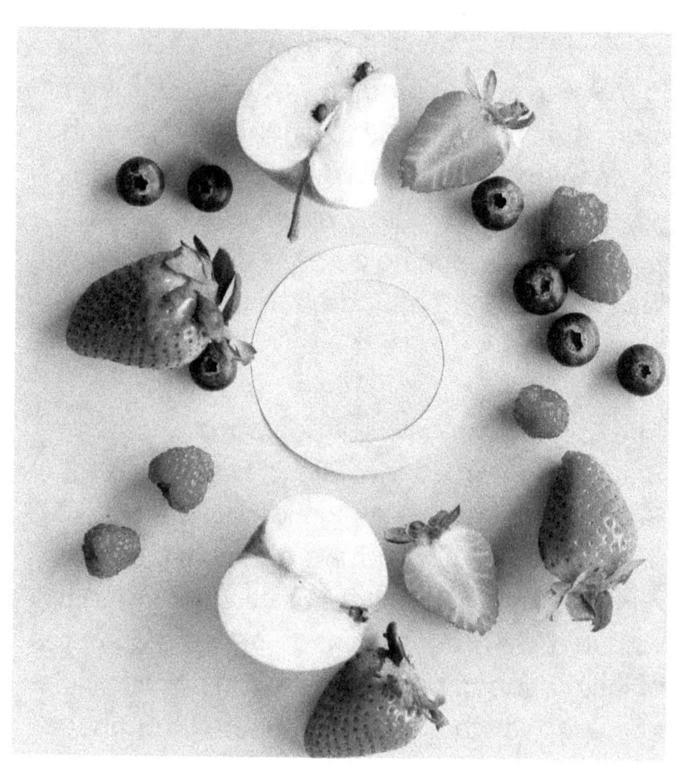

Understanding Blood Sugar and Aging

Understanding the intricate relationship between blood sugar and aging is akin to deciphering the subtle nuances of a well-aged wine. As the years gracefully accumulate, so too does the complexity of our body's mechanisms for regulating blood sugar levels. Let's embark on a journey through the physiological tapestry that intertwines these two aspects.

Physiological Changes:
With the passing of time, our body undergoes various physiological changes. Cells become less responsive to insulin, the hormone crucial for regulating blood sugar. This insulin resistance can lead to elevated blood sugar levels, a common concern in aging individuals.

Impact on Metabolism:
The metabolism, akin to a finely tuned engine, experiences a slowdown. This can affect the body's ability to efficiently process glucose, contributing to fluctuations in blood sugar. Understanding these metabolic shifts becomes paramount in navigating the aging process healthily.

Influence of Lifestyle Factors:
Aging isn't solely determined by biological clocks; lifestyle choices play a pivotal role. Sedentary habits and dietary patterns can exacerbate the challenges of blood sugar regulation. Recognizing how lifestyle intertwines with aging empowers individuals to make informed choices for their well-being.

Role of Inflammation:
Inflammation, a natural response to stress or injury, can escalate with age. Chronic inflammation can impair insulin sensitivity, disrupting the delicate dance of blood sugar balance. Exploring the connection between aging, inflammation, and blood sugar sheds light on proactive measures for health maintenance.

The Gut-Brain Axis:
The gut, often referred to as the "second brain," undergoes changes as we age. This can impact digestion, nutrient absorption, and, consequently, blood sugar regulation. Understanding the symbiotic relationship between the gut and the brain provides insights into holistic approaches for senior health.

Hormonal Fluctuations:
Hormonal changes, a hallmark of aging, can influence blood sugar dynamics.

Fluctuations in hormones such as cortisol and growth hormone can impact insulin sensitivity. A nuanced understanding of these hormonal shifts aids in tailoring strategies for managing blood sugar in seniors.

Genetic Predispositions:
Unraveling the genetic fabric that shapes an individual's predisposition to blood sugar challenges is crucial. Aging often unveils underlying genetic factors that may contribute to the risk of conditions like diabetes. Acknowledging these genetic markers empowers individuals to adopt personalized health strategies.

Importance of Managing Blood Sugar in Seniors

The importance of managing blood sugar in seniors extends far beyond the realm of mere medical diligence; it is a pivotal cornerstone for fostering a vibrant and resilient chapter in the tapestry of aging. Let's delve into the profound significance of this endeavor, recognizing it as a key to unlocking a life rich in vitality and well-being.

Preventing Chronic Conditions:
Effectively managing blood sugar plays a crucial role in preventing chronic conditions, notably Type 2 diabetes. Seniors are often more susceptible to insulin resistance, and by proactively regulating blood sugar levels, they can mitigate the risk of developing long-term health complications.

Preserving Cognitive Function:
The intricate connection between blood sugar levels and cognitive function becomes increasingly apparent in the aging process. Unstable blood sugar can contribute to cognitive decline and an increased risk of conditions like dementia. Managing blood sugar is, therefore, a strategy for preserving mental acuity and cognitive well-being.

Enhancing Cardiovascular Health:
Elevated blood sugar is a significant risk factor for cardiovascular diseases. Seniors who actively manage their blood sugar levels contribute to maintaining heart health, reducing the likelihood of issues such as heart attacks and strokes. This, in turn, fosters a resilient cardiovascular system.

Promoting Energy and Vitality:
Stable blood sugar levels are synonymous with sustained energy and vitality. Seniors who prioritize blood sugar management experience fewer energy fluctuations, enabling them to engage in daily activities with vigor and enthusiasm. This fosters a sense of well-being and an enhanced quality of life.

Supporting Immune Function:
The immune system's efficacy is intricately linked to blood sugar regulation. Seniors with well-managed blood sugar levels bolster their immune function, enhancing their ability to resist infections and illnesses. This becomes especially crucial in maintaining overall health and resilience.

Preventing Complications:
Uncontrolled blood sugar can lead to a cascade of complications, ranging from nerve damage to kidney issues.

Actively managing blood sugar in seniors helps prevent these complications, ensuring a higher quality of life and reducing the burden of medical interventions.

Improving Emotional Well-Being:
The emotional well-being of seniors is profoundly influenced by their physical health. Stable blood sugar levels contribute to a balanced mood and reduced stress levels. Managing blood sugar becomes a tool for promoting emotional resilience and a positive outlook on life.

Empowering Personal Independence:
Seniors who take charge of their blood sugar management are better positioned to maintain personal independence. This self-care aspect fosters a sense of control over one's health, allowing seniors to actively participate in daily activities and maintain a fulfilling lifestyle.

In essence, the importance of managing blood sugar in seniors transcends the boundaries of health; it is a testament to the commitment to living a life brimming with vitality, resilience, and a sense of empowerment. By recognizing the profound impact of blood sugar on various facets of well-being, seniors can embark on a journey towards aging gracefully, with each day unfolding as a celebration of health and life.

CHAPTER ONE

The Senior Health Landscape

The Senior Health Landscape is a panoramic view that encompasses the multifaceted terrain of health and well-being as individuals gracefully transition into their later years. It involves an intricate interplay of physical, mental, and social dimensions, each contributing to the overall tapestry of senior health. Let's explore the various aspects that shape this landscape:

Physical Health:
At the forefront of the Senior Health Landscape is physical well-being. As individuals age, they encounter changes in metabolism, muscle mass, and bone density.

Managing chronic conditions, addressing
mobility issues, and promoting healthy lifestyle
choices become crucial elements in cultivating
a resilient physical health foundation.

Cognitive Well-Being:
Cognitive health is a pivotal component of the
landscape, influencing memory, reasoning, and
overall mental acuity. Seniors navigate the
challenges of maintaining cognitive function,
with a focus on preventing conditions like
dementia. Engaging in mentally stimulating
activities, adopting a brain-healthy diet, and
staying socially active contribute to cognitive
well-being.

Emotional Resilience:
Emotional health plays a significant role in the
Senior Health Landscape. Seniors often face
life transitions, loss of loved ones, and changes
in social roles. Nurturing emotional resilience
involves addressing mental health, managing
stress, and fostering a positive outlook.

Social connections and support networks become vital elements in this emotional journey.

Social Connectivity:
The landscape is enriched by the social fabric woven through the lives of seniors. Maintaining social connections, participating in community activities, and cultivating friendships contribute to a sense of belonging and purpose. Social isolation, conversely, can have detrimental effects on both mental and physical health.

Nutritional Foundations:
Nutrition becomes a cornerstone in the Senior Health Landscape. Addressing dietary needs, ensuring adequate intake of essential nutrients, and managing conditions like malnutrition or obesity are integral components. A well-balanced diet tailored to the unique needs of seniors supports overall health and vitality.

Medical Management:
The landscape encompasses the intricacies of
medical care, involving regular check-ups,
management of chronic conditions, and
adherence to medication regimens. Access to
healthcare services and proactive health
monitoring contribute to a comprehensive
approach in safeguarding senior health.

Physical Activity and Mobility:
Maintaining mobility and incorporating physical
activity into daily routines are critical elements
of the landscape. Seniors benefit from exercise
that enhances balance, flexibility, and strength.
This not only supports physical health but also
contributes to fall prevention and an active
lifestyle.

Preventive Health Measures:
The Senior Health Landscape emphasizes the importance of preventive measures. Immunizations, screenings, and health education play a pivotal role in warding off potential health challenges. Proactive health management allows seniors to age with resilience and minimize the impact of preventable conditions.

In essence, the Senior Health Landscape is a dynamic and interconnected panorama, where each facet contributes to the overall picture of health and well-being. It is a canvas upon which seniors can paint a vibrant and fulfilling journey, navigating the complexities of aging with grace, resilience, and an unwavering commitment to living a life of optimal health.

Common Health Issues in Seniors Related to Blood Sugar

Seniors often face specific health issues related to blood sugar, reflecting the intricate interplay between aging and metabolic changes. Understanding these common health issues is crucial for proactive management and improved overall well-being. Here are some key aspects:

Type 2 Diabetes:
A prevalent concern among seniors is the development or exacerbation of Type 2 diabetes. This condition is characterized by insulin resistance, where the body's cells become less responsive to insulin, leading to elevated blood sugar levels. Seniors are at an increased risk due to age-related changes in metabolism.

Hypoglycemia:
Seniors may experience episodes of low blood sugar (hypoglycemia), especially if they are taking medications for diabetes. Factors such as irregular meal times, medication interactions, or changes in physical activity levels can contribute to hypoglycemic events, posing risks like dizziness, confusion, and fainting.

Hyperglycemia:
On the flip side, hyperglycemia, or high blood sugar levels, is a concern. It can be linked to insulin resistance, inadequate medication management, or dietary choices. Persistent hyperglycemia can lead to complications such as cardiovascular issues, kidney problems, and impaired wound healing.

Cardiovascular Complications:
Elevated blood sugar levels can contribute to cardiovascular complications, a significant concern for seniors. Diabetes increases the risk of heart disease, stroke, and other vascular issues. Managing blood sugar becomes crucial in preventing or mitigating these potentially serious complications.

Neuropathy:
Seniors with uncontrolled blood sugar levels may experience neuropathy, a condition characterized by nerve damage. This can lead to pain, tingling, or numbness in the extremities. Foot care is particularly important as seniors with diabetes are more susceptible to foot-related complications.

Vision Problems:
Diabetes-related eye complications, such as diabetic retinopathy, become more prevalent in seniors. Uncontrolled blood sugar can damage blood vessels in the eyes, leading to vision problems or even blindness. Regular eye exams and blood sugar management are essential for preserving vision.

Kidney Disease:
Seniors with diabetes face an increased risk of kidney disease. Persistent high blood sugar levels can damage the kidneys over time. Regular monitoring of kidney function and adopting lifestyle measures to manage blood sugar are crucial for kidney health.

Cognitive Impacts:
Emerging research suggests a link between diabetes and cognitive decline in seniors. Uncontrolled blood sugar may contribute to conditions like dementia or Alzheimer's disease. Proactive blood sugar management is viewed as a potential protective measure against cognitive impairment.

Understanding and addressing these common health issues related to blood sugar in seniors require a holistic approach. It involves regular medical check-ups, adherence to prescribed medications, maintaining a healthy lifestyle, and staying informed about the potential impacts of blood sugar on various aspects of health. By taking proactive measures, seniors can navigate these challenges with resilience and optimize their overall well-being.

Impact of Diet on Senior Health

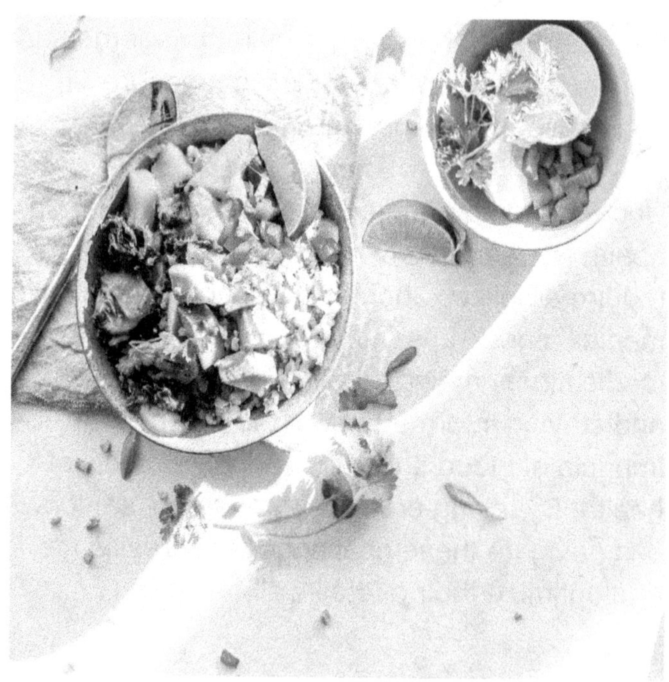

The impact of diet on senior health is profound, influencing not only physical well-being but also cognitive function, immune resilience, and overall quality of life. As individuals age, their nutritional needs evolve, making dietary choices a critical factor in promoting optimal health. Here are key aspects of how diet affects senior health:

Nutrient Density:
Seniors often face a reduction in caloric needs, emphasizing the importance of nutrient-dense foods. A diet rich in vitamins, minerals, and other essential nutrients supports overall health, ensuring seniors meet their nutritional requirements without unnecessary calories.

Bone Health:
Adequate calcium and vitamin D intake is crucial for maintaining bone health in seniors. As bones naturally weaken with age, a diet supporting bone density can help prevent fractures and conditions like osteoporosis.

Heart Health:
Dietary choices significantly impact cardiovascular health. Seniors benefit from a heart-healthy diet low in saturated fats, cholesterol, and sodium. Emphasizing fruits, vegetables, whole grains, and lean proteins contributes to managing blood pressure and reducing the risk of heart disease.

Blood Sugar Management:
For seniors dealing with or at risk of diabetes, managing blood sugar levels through diet is paramount. A balanced and consistent intake of carbohydrates, paired with monitoring portion sizes, aids in preventing spikes or dips in blood sugar.

Cognitive Function:
Emerging research suggests a connection
between diet and cognitive function in seniors.
Antioxidant-rich foods, omega-3 fatty acids,
and a diet low in processed foods may
contribute to cognitive health, potentially
reducing the risk of cognitive decline.

Gut Health:
The gut microbiome plays a vital role in overall
health, including digestion and immune
function. A diet rich in fiber, probiotics, and
prebiotics supports a healthy gut, promoting
nutrient absorption and a robust immune
system.

Weight Management:
Seniors often face changes in metabolism and muscle mass, making weight management a crucial aspect of health. A well-balanced diet that meets nutritional needs while considering calorie intake supports healthy weight maintenance.

Hydration:
Dehydration is a common concern in seniors and can lead to various health issues. Ensuring an adequate intake of fluids, including water and hydrating foods, is vital for maintaining proper bodily functions, especially as the sensation of thirst may decrease with age.

Chronic Disease Prevention and Management:
Dietary choices can impact the prevention and management of chronic conditions common in seniors, such as diabetes, hypertension, and cardiovascular diseases. Adopting a diet aligned with medical recommendations contributes to overall health and well-being.

Social and Emotional Aspects:
Sharing meals and enjoying food in a social context can contribute to emotional well-being. The pleasure of eating, coupled with social interactions, enhances the overall dining experience for seniors, promoting a positive relationship with food.

In essence, the impact of diet on senior health extends far beyond mere sustenance. It is a cornerstone for maintaining vitality, preventing age-related conditions, and optimizing the overall aging process. By embracing a nutritious and well-balanced diet tailored to their unique needs, seniors can proactively nurture their health, fostering a vibrant and fulfilling quality of life.

CHAPTER TWO

Basics of Blood Sugar Regulation

The basics of blood sugar regulation for seniors involve understanding how the body manages glucose, the role of insulin, and the factors that can influence blood sugar levels. As individuals age, the intricacies of this regulation become particularly relevant. Here's an overview of the fundamental elements:

Glucose Metabolism:
Glucose, derived from carbohydrates in the diet, serves as the primary energy source for the body. After consuming food, the digestive system breaks down carbohydrates into glucose, which enters the bloodstream, raising blood sugar levels.

Insulin Function:
Insulin, produced by the pancreas, plays a central role in blood sugar regulation. When blood sugar levels rise after a meal, insulin is released to facilitate the uptake of glucose into cells for energy use or storage. Insulin helps lower blood sugar levels back to a stable range.

Insulin Resistance:
Seniors may experience insulin resistance, a condition where cells become less responsive to insulin. This can lead to elevated blood sugar levels as glucose has difficulty entering cells. Insulin resistance is a common factor in age-related changes in metabolism.

Blood Sugar Levels: Following an overnight fast, blood sugar levels are assessed. It offers a baseline understanding of the body's ability to control blood sugar levels independent of current dietary intake.

Diabetes or insulin resistance may be indicated
by elevated fasting blood sugar.

Postprandial Blood Sugar:
Postprandial blood sugar levels are measured
after meals. Seniors may experience
challenges in regulating postprandial blood
sugar due to factors such as slower digestion
and reduced insulin sensitivity. Monitoring
these levels helps assess how the body
responds to dietary choices.

Role of the Liver:
The liver plays a crucial role in blood sugar
regulation. It stores glucose as glycogen and
releases it into the bloodstream between meals
to maintain stable blood sugar levels. In
seniors, age-related changes in liver function
can impact this process.

Dietary Factors:
The composition and timing of meals significantly influence blood sugar regulation. Seniors benefit from a balanced diet that includes complex carbohydrates, fiber, and lean proteins. Consistent meal timing and portion control are essential for managing blood sugar levels.

Physical Activity:
Regular physical activity enhances insulin sensitivity and helps control blood sugar levels. Seniors should engage in exercise appropriate for their fitness level, incorporating both aerobic activities and strength training to support overall metabolic health.

Medication Management:
Some seniors may require medications to help manage blood sugar levels, especially if they have diabetes.

Adherence to prescribed medications and regular communication with healthcare providers are crucial for effective blood sugar control.

Regular Monitoring:
Seniors should monitor their blood sugar levels regularly, especially if they have diabetes or are at risk of developing it. Regular monitoring provides insights into how lifestyle factors, diet, and medications impact blood sugar levels.

Understanding the basics of blood sugar regulation empowers seniors to make informed decisions about their lifestyle, diet, and overall health. Proactive management, in collaboration with healthcare professionals, ensures a balanced and stable blood sugar environment, contributing to optimal well-being in the senior years.

How the Body Manages Blood Sugar

As individuals age, the body undergoes changes in the way it manages blood sugar. Understanding these age-related shifts is crucial for seniors to proactively support their health. Here's an overview of how the body manages blood sugar in seniors:

Insulin Sensitivity Changes:
Seniors often experience a decline in insulin sensitivity, a phenomenon where cells become less responsive to insulin. This can result in higher blood sugar levels as the body struggles to efficiently utilize glucose for energy.

Pancreatic Function:
The pancreas, responsible for producing insulin, may exhibit changes in function with age. The production and release of insulin might become less efficient, impacting the body's ability to regulate blood sugar promptly.

Liver Function:
The liver plays a crucial role in blood sugar regulation. It stores glucose as glycogen and releases it into the bloodstream between meals to maintain stable blood sugar levels. However, age-related changes in liver function can affect this process, leading to variations in blood sugar.

Slower Digestion:
Aging can contribute to slower digestion, affecting the rate at which carbohydrates are broken down into glucose. This slower process may lead to prolonged postprandial (after-meal) increases in blood sugar.

Decreased Physical Activity:
Seniors may experience reduced physical activity levels, impacting the body's ability to efficiently use glucose. Regular exercise is essential for enhancing insulin sensitivity and promoting optimal blood sugar management.

Changes in Body Composition:
Changes in body composition, such as decreased muscle mass and increased fat mass, can affect how the body processes glucose. Muscle tissue is a significant consumer of glucose, and reductions in muscle mass may contribute to insulin resistance.

Hormonal Fluctuations:
Hormonal changes associated with aging, such as alterations in growth hormone and cortisol levels, can influence blood sugar regulation. These fluctuations may contribute to insulin resistance and impact overall metabolic health.

Medication Considerations:
Some seniors may be on medications that affect blood sugar levels. It's crucial for seniors to work closely with healthcare providers to ensure that prescribed medications align with their changing physiological needs and contribute to effective blood sugar control.

Dietary Adjustments:
Seniors benefit from dietary adjustments that consider changes in metabolism and insulin sensitivity. Emphasizing a well-balanced diet with controlled portion sizes, complex carbohydrates, and adequate protein is essential for supporting blood sugar management.

Regular Monitoring:
Regular monitoring of blood sugar levels is particularly important for seniors, especially those with diabetes or insulin resistance. This monitoring provides valuable insights into how the body responds to dietary choices, physical activity, and medication.

In summary, the aging process introduces a range of factors that impact how the body manages blood sugar. Seniors can navigate these changes by adopting a holistic approach that includes lifestyle modifications, dietary adjustments, regular physical activity, and close collaboration with healthcare professionals to optimize blood sugar control and overall metabolic health.

Factors Affecting Blood Sugar Levels in Seniors

Several factors can influence blood sugar levels in seniors, and understanding these factors is crucial for managing and maintaining optimal blood sugar control. Here are key elements that can affect blood sugar levels in seniors:

Insulin Resistance:
Seniors often experience insulin resistance, where cells become less responsive to insulin. This condition impairs the body's ability to efficiently use glucose, leading to elevated blood sugar levels.

Changes in Metabolism:
Aging is associated with changes in metabolism, including a decrease in basal metabolic rate. This can impact how the body processes and utilizes glucose, potentially leading to fluctuations in blood sugar levels.

Physical Activity Levels:
Reduced physical activity, common in seniors, can contribute to insulin resistance and affect blood sugar regulation. Engaging in regular exercise helps enhance insulin sensitivity and supports better blood sugar control.

Dietary Choices:
The composition of meals and the timing of food intake significantly influence blood sugar levels. Seniors should focus on a well-balanced diet, paying attention to portion sizes, and incorporating complex carbohydrates, fiber, and lean proteins to mitigate spikes in blood sugar.

Medications:
Certain medications, including those prescribed for conditions unrelated to blood sugar, can impact glucose levels. Seniors should be aware of the potential effects of their medications on blood sugar and work closely with healthcare providers to adjust treatment plans if needed.

Stress Levels:
Stress can trigger the release of hormones such as cortisol, which may lead to increased blood sugar levels. Seniors should implement stress-management techniques, such as meditation or relaxation exercises, to mitigate the impact on blood sugar.

Sleep Quality:
Poor sleep or irregular sleep patterns can affect blood sugar regulation. Seniors should prioritize good sleep hygiene to support overall health, including stable blood sugar levels.

Hydration Status:
Dehydration can lead to higher blood sugar
concentrations. Seniors should ensure they
stay adequately hydrated to support proper
bodily functions, including the regulation of
blood sugar.

Underlying Health Conditions:
Certain health conditions, such as infections or
inflammation, can influence blood sugar levels.
Seniors with chronic illnesses should be
vigilant about managing their overall health to
minimize the impact on blood sugar.

Hormonal Changes:
Hormonal fluctuations associated with aging,
such as changes in estrogen and testosterone
levels, can affect blood sugar control.
Understanding and addressing these hormonal
changes are essential for maintaining optimal
blood sugar levels.

Genetic Predisposition:
Genetic factors can play a role in blood sugar regulation. Seniors with a family history of diabetes or related conditions may have a higher risk, emphasizing the importance of proactive management and monitoring.

In summary, a holistic approach to blood sugar management in seniors involves addressing multiple factors, including lifestyle choices, medication management, stress levels, and overall health. Regular monitoring and collaboration with healthcare professionals are essential to tailor strategies that support stable blood sugar levels and promote overall well-being.

CHAPTER THREE

Senior-Friendly Nutritional Guidelines

Senior-friendly nutritional guidelines encompass various aspects to address the changing dietary needs of older adults. Here's a more detailed breakdown:

Caloric Intake:

Adjust caloric intake based on individual factors such as activity level, metabolism, and health conditions.
Balance energy consumption with expenditure to prevent weight-related issues.

Nutrient-Dense Foods:
Prioritize nutrient-dense foods rich in vitamins, minerals, and antioxidants.
Include a variety of fruits, vegetables, whole grains, lean proteins, and healthy fats to meet essential nutrient requirements.

Calcium and Vitamin D:
Emphasize calcium and vitamin D intake for bone health and to reduce the risk of osteoporosis.
Dairy products, leafy greens, fortified cereals, and fatty fish are good sources.

Fiber Intake:
Ensure sufficient fiber intake to support digestive health and prevent constipation.
Include whole grains, fruits, vegetables, legumes, and nuts in the diet.

Hydration:
Encourage proper hydration, as older adults may have a reduced sense of thirst.
Water, herbal teas, and hydrating foods like fruits and vegetables contribute to overall fluid intake.

Maintaining sufficient protein consumption is necessary to support muscular mass, which decreases with aging.
Add plant-based protein sources, chicken, fish, eggs, dairy, and lean meats.

Addressing Dental Issues:
Choose softer or easily chewable foods to accommodate potential dental problems.
Adequate dental care and regular check-ups are essential for maintaining oral health.

Appetite Considerations:
Be mindful of potential reduced appetite and adjust portion sizes accordingly.
Encourage regular, smaller meals and snacks to ensure adequate nutrient intake.

Managing Medication Interactions:
Consider potential interactions between medications and certain nutrients.
Consult healthcare professionals to adapt the diet based on medication requirements.

Cultural and Individual Preferences:
Respect cultural preferences and individual dietary choices.
Tailor recommendations to accommodate personal tastes while meeting nutritional needs.

Portion control is a technique that can help you manage your weight and stop overeating. Reduce the size of your dishes and bowls to promote attentive eating.

Regular Meals:
Establish a routine with regular meals to provide stability and support nutritional intake. Avoid skipping meals and encourage a balanced distribution of nutrients throughout the day.

These guidelines aim to promote overall well-being in older adults, ensuring they receive the necessary nutrients for optimal health while addressing specific challenges associated with aging.

Essential Nutrients for Seniors

For seniors focusing on maintaining blood sugar levels, certain essential nutrients play a crucial role in supporting a balanced and stable metabolism. Here are key nutrients with relevance to a blood sugar-friendly diet:

Fiber: Promotes improved blood sugar regulation by helping to slow down the absorption of sugar.
present in fruits, vegetables, whole grains, legumes, and nuts.

Magnesium: Enhances glucose regulation and helps modulate insulin sensitivity.
Nuts, seeds, leafy greens, and whole grains are examples of sources.

Chromium:
Supports insulin action, assisting in glucose metabolism.
Present in small amounts in meats, whole grains, and some fruits and vegetables.

Vitamin D:
Plays a role in insulin sensitivity.
Sun exposure, fatty fish, fortified foods, and supplements are sources.

Omega-3 Fatty Acids:
May improve insulin sensitivity and reduce inflammation.
Fatty fish (salmon, mackerel), flaxseeds, chia seeds, and walnuts are sources.

Protein: By reducing the rate at which glucose is absorbed, it helps to balance blood sugar levels.
Good options include fish, chicken, lentils, dairy products, and plant-based proteins.

Vitamin C:
Antioxidant properties may benefit blood sugar control.
Found in citrus fruits, berries, and various vegetables.

Zinc:
Supports insulin production and may contribute to better blood sugar regulation.
Present in meat, dairy, nuts, seeds, and whole grains.

Vanadium:
Some studies suggest a potential role in
improving insulin sensitivity.
Found in mushrooms, shellfish, and certain
vegetables.

B Vitamins (B6, B12, Folate):
Play a role in carbohydrate metabolism and
may aid in blood sugar control.
Found in various foods, including meats, dairy,
leafy greens, and legumes.

Cinnamon:
While not a nutrient, cinnamon may help
improve insulin sensitivity.
Can be added to foods or consumed as a
supplement (consult with a healthcare
professional).

Water:
Staying hydrated is essential for overall health,
including blood sugar regulation.
Water and herbal teas are excellent choices.

Crafting a Balanced Diet for Blood Sugar Management

Crafting a balanced diet for effective blood sugar management involves thoughtful consideration of nutrient composition, meal timing, and portion control. Here's a guide to help achieve and maintain stable blood sugar levels:

Stress Complex carbs: As your main sources of carbs, go for whole grains, legumes, and vegetables.
Give up processed carbohydrates and sugary meals in favor of lentils, brown rice, quinoa, and sweet potatoes.

Include High-Fiber Foods:
Prioritize fiber-rich foods to slow down the absorption of glucose.
Incorporate fruits, vegetables, whole grains, nuts, and seeds into your meals.

Moderate Portion Sizes: To prevent overindulging and reduce calorie intake, practice portion management.
Reduce the size of your dishes and bowls to promote attentive eating.

Combine Proteins and Healthy Fats:
Pair lean proteins (chicken, fish, tofu) with healthy fats (avocado, nuts, olive oil) to enhance satiety and regulate blood sugar.
Avoid excessive saturated and trans fats found in processed and fried foods.

Select Low-Glycemic Index Foods: To avoid sharp spikes in blood sugar, choose foods with a lower glycemic index.
Legumes, most fruits, and non-starchy vegetables are a few examples.

Regular Meal Timing: To control blood sugar levels, create a regular meal routine.
Try to eat three well-balanced meals a day, and if necessary, add healthy snacks.

Include Omega-3 Fatty Acids:
Incorporate fatty fish (salmon, mackerel), flaxseeds, and walnuts for their omega-3 content, which may improve insulin sensitivity.

Reduce Added Sugars: Cut back on processed meals, sweetened beverages, and desserts.
To find hidden sugars, read labels carefully and use natural sweeteners sparingly.

Remain Hydrated: To promote general health and hydration, sip copious amounts of water throughout the day.
Choose water, herbal teas, or infused water in place of sugary drinks as often as possible.

Frequent Physical Activity: Exercise on a regular basis to enhance insulin sensitivity and to support general health.
Speak with medical experts to create an appropriate workout regimen.

Monitor Blood Sugar Levels:
Regularly check blood sugar levels to understand how dietary choices impact glucose levels.
Adjust the diet based on these observations and consult healthcare professionals for guidance.
Consult with Healthcare

Professionals:
Work closely with healthcare providers, including a registered dietitian, to create a personalized meal plan based on individual health needs and goals.

Crafting a balanced diet for blood sugar management involves a holistic approach that combines nutrient-dense foods, mindful eating, and lifestyle factors. Individualized guidance from healthcare professionals ensures a plan tailored to specific health conditions and requirements.

CHAPTER FOUR

The Role of Exercise for Seniors

Exercise plays a crucial role in the blood sugar solution for seniors, contributing to improved glucose control and overall health. Here are key aspects of the role of exercise for seniors in managing blood sugar:

Enhanced Insulin Sensitivity:
Regular physical activity improves insulin sensitivity, allowing cells to use insulin more effectively.
This can help seniors manage blood sugar levels more efficiently.

Glucose Regulation:
Exercise helps regulate blood sugar by
increasing the uptake of glucose by muscles
for energy during physical activity.
This effect continues even after exercise,
contributing to more stable blood sugar levels.

Weight Management:
Regular exercise supports weight maintenance
or weight loss, which is crucial for seniors with
diabetes or those at risk.
Maintaining a healthy weight positively impacts
insulin sensitivity and overall metabolic health.

Muscle Health:
Strength training exercises help preserve and
build muscle mass, which is especially
important for seniors as they may experience
age-related muscle loss.
Muscles play a significant role in glucose
uptake, and maintaining muscle health aids in
blood sugar management.

Improved Blood Lipid Profile:
Regular physical activity can positively impact cholesterol levels, reducing the risk of cardiovascular complications associated with diabetes.

Stress Reduction:
Exercise is known to reduce stress levels, which can indirectly benefit blood sugar control.
Stress hormones can influence blood sugar, and managing stress through exercise helps mitigate this impact.

Cardiovascular Health:
Exercise contributes to cardiovascular health, reducing the risk of heart disease, a common concern for seniors with diabetes.
Improved circulation supports the delivery of oxygen and nutrients to cells.

Improved Mental Health and Mood:
Engaging in physical activity generates
endorphins, which elevate mood and lower the
likelihood of anxiety and despair.
Sustaining mental well-being is crucial for
general wellbeing and following a healthy
lifestyle.

Joint Health and Flexibility:
Engaging in activities that promote joint health
and flexibility is important for seniors.
Low-impact exercises, such as swimming or
gentle yoga, can be suitable options.

Balance and Fall Prevention:
Certain exercises, including balance and
stability training, can help prevent falls, which
is crucial for older adults.
Reducing the risk of injuries is particularly
important for those with diabetes, as
complications from falls can be severe.

Individualized Approach:
Consideration of individual health conditions
and fitness levels is essential when prescribing
exercise for seniors.
Consultation with healthcare professionals and
personalized exercise plans ensure safety and
effectiveness.

In summary, regular and appropriate exercise
is a key component of the blood sugar solution
for seniors. It offers a range of benefits, from
improved glucose control to enhanced overall
health and well-being. As always, seniors
should consult with healthcare providers before
starting a new exercise regimen, especially if
they have pre-existing health conditions.

Tailoring Exercise Programs for Older Adults

Tailoring exercise programs for older adults involves considering their unique needs, health conditions, and fitness levels. Here's a guide on how to customize exercise programs for this demographic:

Health Assessment:
Begin with a thorough health assessment, considering existing medical conditions, mobility issues, and any limitations. Consultation with healthcare professionals helps identify potential concerns and ensures safety.

Individualized Approach:
Recognize the diversity among older adults and tailor programs to individual abilities, preferences, and goals.
Consider factors such as fitness level, chronic conditions, and any previous injuries.

Low-Impact Activities:
Choose low-impact exercises to reduce stress
on joints and minimize the risk of injuries.
Options include walking, swimming, cycling,
and low-impact aerobics.

Strength Training:
Include strength training exercises to maintain
or build muscle mass, essential for overall
health.
Use resistance bands, light weights, or
bodyweight exercises focusing on major
muscle groups.

Flexibility and Balance:
Incorporate activities that improve flexibility and
balance, crucial for preventing falls.
Yoga, tai chi, and simple stretching routines are
beneficial.

Gradual Progression:
Introduce exercises gradually, allowing older adults to adapt and avoid overexertion. Progression should be gradual, considering both intensity and duration.

Functional Movements:
Emphasize exercises that mimic daily activities to enhance functional fitness.
For example, incorporating squats, lunges, and reaching exercises improves overall mobility.

Regular Cardiovascular Exercise:
Include aerobic exercises to promote cardiovascular health.
Aim for at least 150 minutes of moderate-intensity exercise per week, or as recommended by healthcare professionals.

Supervision and Instruction:
Provide clear instructions and, if possible, supervised sessions to ensure proper form and technique.
Supervision can enhance safety and effectiveness, especially for those new to exercise.

Adaptations for Mobility Issues:
Modify exercises to accommodate mobility issues, using chairs or other support as needed.
Water-based activities can be particularly beneficial for those with joint concerns.

Social Engagement:
Encourage group exercises or classes to foster social connections, which contribute to overall well-being.
Social engagement can enhance motivation and adherence to exercise routines.

Regular Reassessment:
Periodically reassess fitness levels and adjust the exercise program accordingly.
Adaptations may be necessary based on changes in health or functional abilities.

Consideration of Chronic Conditions:
Tailor exercises to accommodate specific chronic conditions, such as arthritis, diabetes, or heart disease.
Coordination with healthcare professionals ensures a safe and effective approach.

Customizing exercise programs for older adults involves a thoughtful and holistic approach, recognizing their unique needs and capabilities. Collaboration between healthcare providers, fitness professionals, and the individuals themselves is key to developing successful and sustainable exercise routines.

Benefits of Physical Activity in Blood Sugar Control

Engaging in regular physical activity offers numerous benefits for blood sugar control, particularly for individuals with diabetes or those at risk of developing the condition. Here are key advantages:

Improved Insulin Sensitivity:
Regular exercise enhances the body's ability to use insulin effectively, improving insulin sensitivity.
This allows cells to take up and utilize glucose more efficiently, leading to better blood sugar control.

Glucose Regulation:
Physical activity helps regulate blood sugar
levels by increasing the uptake of glucose by
muscles during and after exercise.
This reduces the overall concentration of
glucose in the bloodstream.

Weight Management:
Exercise contributes to weight loss or
maintenance, which is crucial for blood sugar
control.
Maintaining a healthy weight improves insulin
sensitivity and reduces the risk of insulin
resistance.

Increased Glucose Uptake by Muscles:
Muscles act as a major reservoir for glucose
uptake during physical activity.
Regular exercise increases the capacity of
muscles to take up and utilize glucose,
reducing circulating blood glucose levels.

Reduced Insulin Resistance:
Insulin resistance, a common issue in type 2 diabetes, is mitigated through regular exercise. Exercise helps overcome resistance, allowing insulin to regulate blood sugar more effectively.

Enhanced Post-Meal Glucose Control:
Physical activity has been shown to lower post-meal glucose levels.
Including short walks after meals can be particularly beneficial in controlling blood sugar spikes.

Cardiovascular Health:
Exercise supports cardiovascular health, reducing the risk of heart disease, a common complication of diabetes.
Improved circulation enhances the delivery of oxygen and nutrients to cells, including those involved in glucose metabolism.

Reduction of Abdominal Fat:
Regular exercise helps reduce abdominal fat, which is associated with insulin resistance. Targeting visceral fat contributes to better blood sugar control.

Lowering A1c Levels:
A1c levels, which provide an average of blood sugar levels over time, can be positively influenced by regular physical activity. Consistent exercise is linked to lower A1c levels in individuals with diabetes.

Stress Reduction:
Physical activity is effective in reducing stress levels, which can impact blood sugar control. Stress hormones can elevate blood sugar, and exercise provides a natural way to alleviate stress.

Improved Lipid Profile:
Exercise positively influences cholesterol
levels, reducing the risk of cardiovascular
complications associated with diabetes.
Improved lipid profiles contribute to overall
cardiovascular health.

Improved Mental Health and Mood: Exercise
produces endorphins, which lift the spirits and
lower the risk of anxiety and despair.
Adherence to good lifestyle choices, such as
blood sugar regulation and food, is supported
by mental well-being.

CHAPTER FIVE

Meal Planning and Recipes

Meal planning for a blood sugar-friendly diet for seniors involves selecting nutrient-dense foods and controlling carbohydrate intake. Here's a simple guide:

Lean Proteins: Opt for lean protein sources like chicken, turkey, fish, eggs, and tofu. These help stabilize blood sugar levels and provide essential nutrients.

Non-Starchy Vegetables: Include a variety of non-starchy vegetables such as leafy greens, broccoli, cauliflower, and bell peppers. These are high in fiber and low in carbohydrates.

Whole Grains: Refined grains should be avoided in favor of whole grains like quinoa, brown rice, and oats. They reduce blood sugar increases by releasing glucose more gradually.

Healthy Fats: Include foods like avocados, almonds, seeds, and olive oil that are high in healthy fats. These may aid in blood sugar regulation and satiety.

Portion Control: Be mindful of serving amounts to prevent overindulging, which may raise blood sugar levels. To visually regulate portion proportions, use smaller plates.

Limit Sugars and Processed Foods: Minimize the intake of added sugars and processed foods, as they can cause rapid spikes in blood sugar. Choose whole, unprocessed foods whenever possible.

Sample Meal Ideas:

Breakfast:
Omelet with vegetables and a slice of whole-grain toast.
Greek yogurt with berries and a handful of nuts.

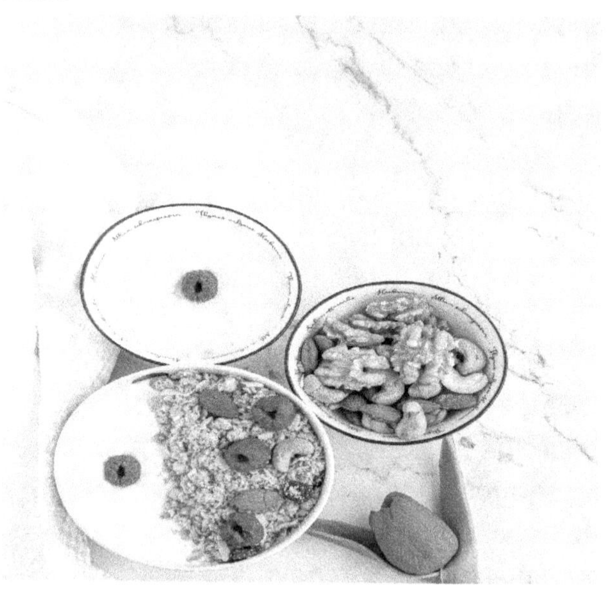

Lunch consists of grilled chicken salad topped
with cherry tomatoes, mixed greens, and
vinaigrette dressing.
quinoa dish with roasted veggies and a protein
serving that is lean.

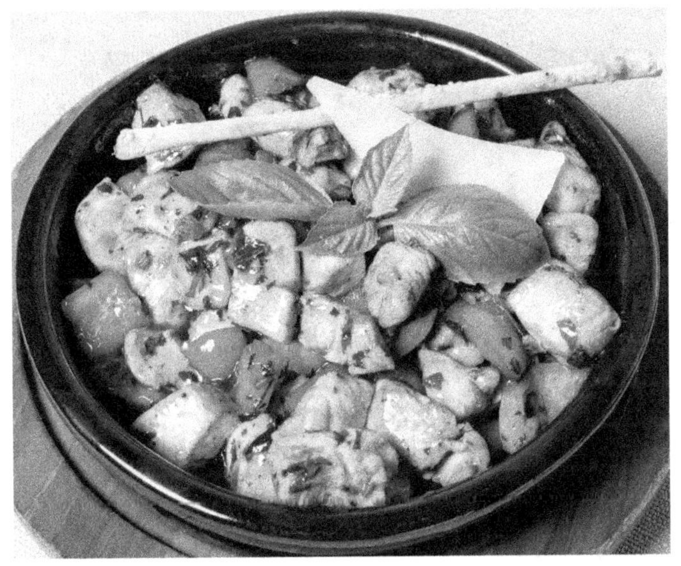

Dinner:
Baked fish with lemon and herbs, steamed broccoli, and quinoa.
Stir-fried tofu with colorful vegetables and brown rice.

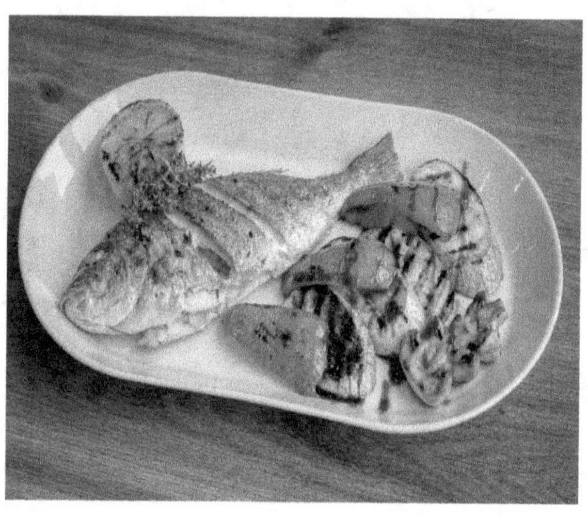

Snacks:
Raw vegetable sticks with hummus.
A small handful of almonds or walnuts.

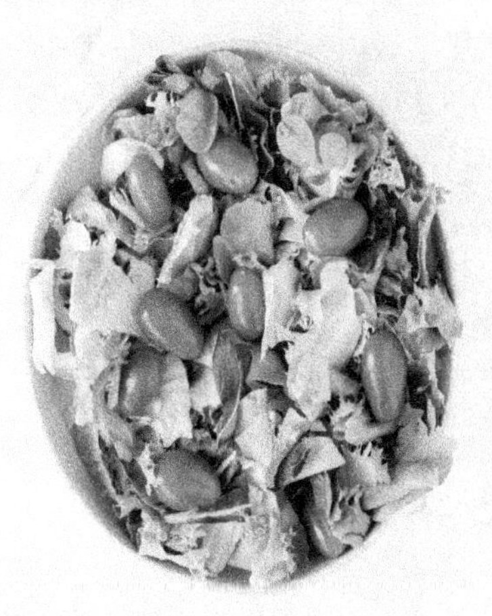

Remember to consult with a healthcare professional or a nutritionist to tailor the plan to specific needs. Regular monitoring of blood sugar levels is crucial for adjusting the diet accordingly.

Sample Meal plans for Seniors

Sample meal plans for seniors focusing on blood sugar control typically include balanced meals with a mix of lean proteins, whole grains, healthy fats, and plenty of vegetables. Here's a sample:

Mid-Morning Snack:
Greek yogurt with sliced almonds
Apple slices.

Lunch:
Grilled chicken salad with mixed greens, cherry tomatoes, cucumbers, and olive oil vinaigrette
Quinoa or brown rice on the side
Water or herbal tea.

Afternoon Snack:
Carrot and cucumber sticks with hummus
A small handful of nuts.

Dinner:
Baked or grilled salmon
Steamed broccoli and cauliflower
Sweet potato or quinoa
Sparkling water with a splash of lemon.

Evening Snack (if needed):
Cottage cheese with a few berries
It's important to note that individual dietary
needs may vary, and consulting with a
healthcare professional or a registered dietitian
can help tailor a meal plan specifically for
someone's health condition and preferences.

Healthy and Delicious Recipes for Blood Sugar Control

1 Grilled Chicken and Vegetable Skewers:

Ingredients:
Chicken breast, cut into cubes
Cherry tomatoes
Bell peppers, various colors, chopped into chunks
Zucchini, sliced
Red onion, cut into wedges
Olive oil
Garlic powder, paprika, salt, and pepper for seasoning.

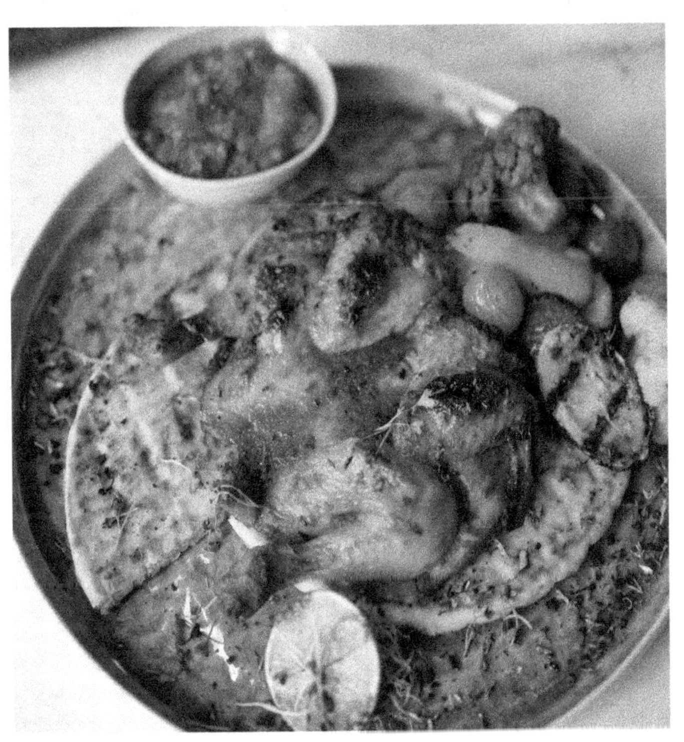

Instructions:
Preheat the grill or oven to medium-high heat.
In a bowl, mix the chicken cubes with olive oil,
garlic powder, paprika, salt, and pepper.
Thread the marinated chicken and vegetables
onto skewers, alternating for a colorful mix.
Grill or bake the skewers until the chicken is
cooked through and the vegetables are tender.
Accompany with quinoa or brown rice on the
side.

2 Quinoa Salad with Chickpeas and Vegetables:

Ingredients:
Cooked quinoa
Canned chickpeas, drained and rinsed
Cherry tomatoes, halved
Cucumber, diced
Red onion, finely chopped
Feta cheese (optional)
Olive oil and lemon juice for dressing
Fresh herbs like parsley or mint
Salt and pepper to taste.

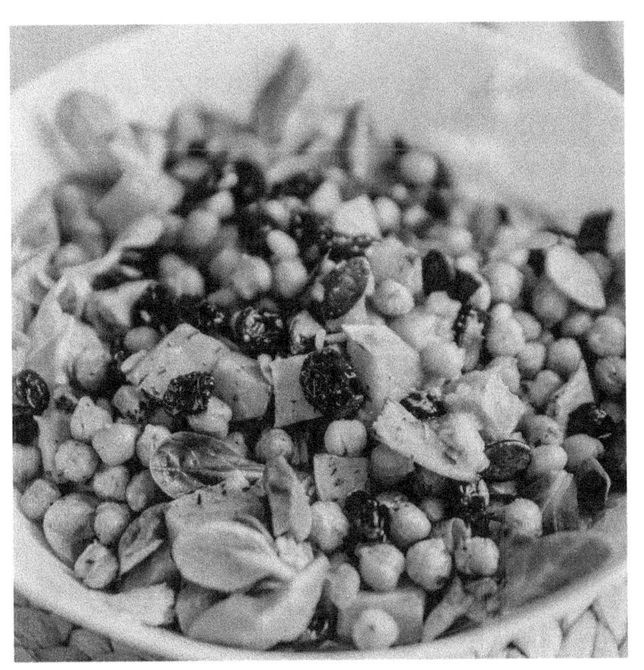

Instructions: Combine cooked quinoa, chickpeas, cucumber, red onion, and cherry tomatoes in a big bowl.

For the salad's dressing, drizzle some lemon juice and olive oil over it.

Gently toss the salad to combine all of the ingredients.

If preferred, garnish with fresh herbs and add feta cheese.

To taste, add salt and pepper for seasoning.

To bring out the flavors, refrigerate for a bit before serving.

These dishes offer a healthy balance of nutrients for blood sugar regulation since they include lean proteins, whole grains, and lots of vegetables. Always adjust recipes to suit dietary requirements and personal preferences.

3 Baked Salmon with Asparagus:

Ingredients:
Salmon filets
Fresh asparagus spears
Lemon slices
Olive oil
Garlic, minced
Dill, chopped
Salt and pepper to taste

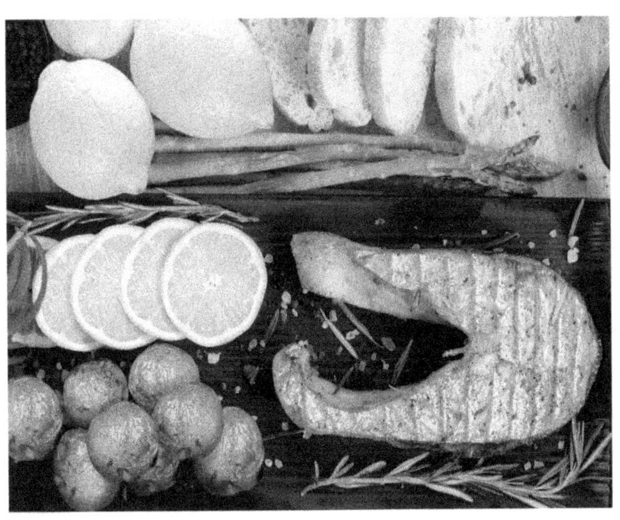

Directions: Preheat the oven to 400°F (200°C). Arrange the asparagus spears around the salmon filets. Drizzle the salmon and asparagus with olive oil. Season the salmon with salt, pepper, minced garlic, and dill. Top the salmon with the lemon slices. Bake for 15 to 20 minutes, or until the salmon is cooked through and flakes easily.

4 Turkey and Vegetable Stir-Fry:

Ingredients:
Ground turkey or turkey breast, thinly sliced
Broccoli florets
Bell peppers, sliced
Snap peas
Garlic, minced
Low-sodium soy sauce
Sesame oil
Ginger, grated
Brown rice or cauliflower rice.

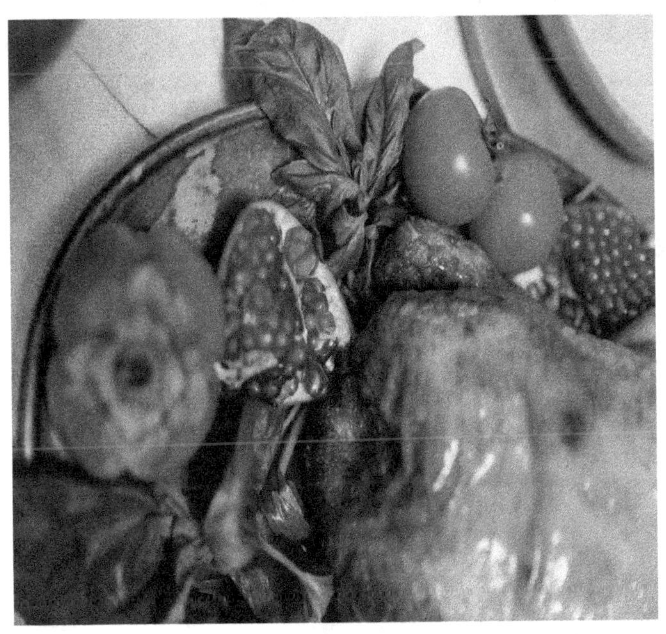

Instructions:
In a wok or large skillet, heat sesame oil and
sauté minced garlic and grated ginger.
Add turkey slices and cook until browned.
Add broccoli, bell peppers, and snap peas to
the wok. Stir-fry until vegetables are
crisp-tender.
Pour in low-sodium soy sauce and continue to
stir-fry for a few minutes.
Serve over brown rice or cauliflower rice.

5 Berry and Greek Yogurt Parfait:

Ingredients:
Greek yogurt
Mixed berries (strawberries, blueberries,
raspberries)
Almonds or walnuts, chopped
Honey (optional)

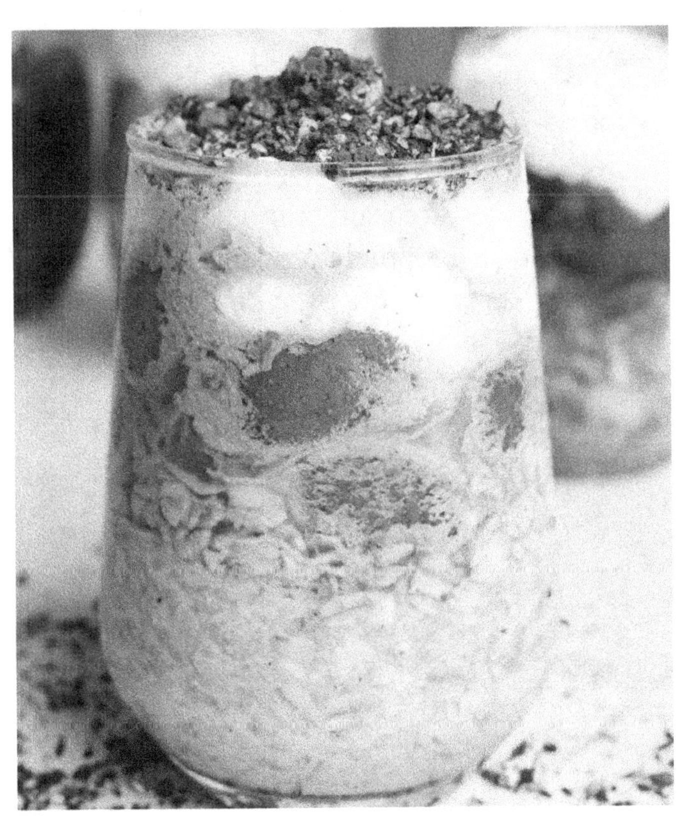

These recipes emphasize lean proteins, vegetables, and healthy fats, making them suitable for controlling blood sugar levels. Modify portion sizes based on individual dietary needs and preferences. Instructions: Layer Greek yogurt with mixed berries in a glass or bowl. Sprinkle chopped nuts on top for added crunch. Drizzle with honey, if desired, for sweetness. Repeat the layers and create an eye-catching parfait.

CHAPTER SIX

Lifestyle Changes for Improved Blood Sugar

Lifestyle changes play a crucial role in managing and improving blood sugar levels. Here are some key lifestyle changes that can contribute to better blood sugar control:

Healthy Eating Habits:
Embrace a balanced diet rich in whole grains, lean proteins, healthy fats, and plenty of fruits and vegetables.
Monitor portion sizes to avoid overeating and maintain a consistent meal schedule.

Frequent Exercise: Take part in regular physical activity, which should include strength training as well as aerobic exercises like swimming, jogging, or walking.
Try to get in at least 150 minutes a week of moderate-to-intense exercise.

Weight Management:
Maintain a healthy weight as excess body weight, especially around the abdomen, can contribute to insulin resistance.
Consult with healthcare professionals or dietitians for personalized weight management plans.

Understanding how to effectively manage stress is crucial since long-term stress can have an impact on blood sugar levels.
Stay hydrated by drinking plenty of water throughout the day.
Limit the consumption of sugary beverages and opt for water, herbal tea, or unsweetened drinks.

Stress Management:
Practice stress-reducing activities such as meditation, deep breathing, yoga, or mindfulness.
Chronic stress can affect blood sugar levels, so finding effective stress management techniques is important.

Sufficient Sleep: Make sure you obtain seven to nine hours of good sleep every night.
Sleep deprivation can interfere with insulin sensitivity and impact blood sugar control.

Regular Monitoring:
Regularly monitor blood sugar levels as advised by healthcare professionals.
Keep a log to track patterns and adjust lifestyle choices accordingly.

Limit Processed Foods: Cut back on refined carbs, sugary snacks, and processed foods. Eat whole, unprocessed foods to help keep blood sugar levels stable.

Quit Smoking:
If applicable, quit smoking, as it can contribute to insulin resistance and increase the risk of complications associated with diabetes.

Regular Health Check-ups:
Schedule regular check-ups with healthcare providers to monitor overall health, including blood pressure, cholesterol levels, and kidney function.

Stress Management for Seniors

Stress management is crucial for seniors to maintain overall well-being and can be approached through various techniques. Here are some stress management strategies tailored for seniors:

Mindfulness and Meditation:
Engage in mindfulness practices, such as meditation or deep-breathing exercises, to promote relaxation and reduce stress.

Gentle Exercise:
Incorporate gentle exercises like walking, tai chi, or yoga into the routine, as they can help alleviate stress and improve mood.

Hobbies and Leisure Activities:
Pursue hobbies and activities that bring joy and relaxation, whether it's reading, gardening, painting, or listening to music.

Social Connections:
Maintain social connections with friends and family. Regular interactions can provide emotional support and a sense of belonging.

Time Management:
Prioritize tasks and manage time effectively. Breaking tasks into smaller, manageable steps can reduce feelings of being overwhelmed.

Relaxation Techniques:
Explore relaxation techniques such as progressive muscle relaxation or guided imagery to ease tension and promote a sense of calm.

Healthy Sleep Habits:
Establish and maintain a regular sleep routine.
Quality sleep is essential for managing stress
and overall well-being.

Limiting News Exposure:
Minimize exposure to distressing news and
focus on positive and uplifting information to
avoid unnecessary stress.

Nutrition:
Maintain a balanced diet with nutritious foods,
as proper nutrition can influence both physical
and mental health.

Adequate Hydration:
Stay hydrated by drinking enough water, as
dehydration can contribute to stress and
fatigue.

Adapting Expectations:
Be realistic about expectations and recognize that it's okay to ask for help when needed.

Nature and Fresh Air:
Spend time outdoors in nature, whether it's a short walk in the park or simply enjoying fresh air on a porch. Nature has a calming effect.

Volunteer Work:
Engage in volunteer activities or community service, fostering a sense of purpose and connection.

Importance of Adequate Sleep

Adequate sleep is integral to maintaining blood sugar levels and is particularly important in the context of managing and preventing issues related to blood sugar, such as diabetes. Here are key reasons highlighting the importance of sufficient sleep for a blood sugar solution:

Insulin Sensitivity:
Adequate sleep supports insulin sensitivity, allowing cells to effectively respond to insulin. This helps regulate blood sugar levels by facilitating the uptake of glucose into cells.

Glucose Metabolism:
During deep sleep, the body undergoes important processes related to glucose metabolism and insulin regulation. Disruptions in these processes can lead to insulin resistance and elevated blood sugar.

Hormonal Balance:
Sleep influences various hormones, including those involved in blood sugar regulation. Imbalances in hormones like cortisol and growth hormone, which occur with inadequate sleep, can lead to glucose dysregulation.

Appetite Control:
Lack of sleep can disrupt the balance of hormones that control appetite, leading to increased cravings for high-calorie and sugary foods. This can contribute to overeating and weight gain, both of which impact blood sugar levels.

Stress Reduction:
Sufficient sleep contributes to stress reduction, as chronic stress can elevate cortisol levels and negatively impact blood sugar regulation. Quality sleep promotes a more balanced stress response.

Energy Balance: A good night's sleep promotes an ideal energy balance, which in turn supports exercise and physical activity. It needs regular exercise to effectively control blood sugar levels.

Control of Inflammation: Extended sleep loss can lead to an increase in the body's inflammatory response. Diabetes mellitus and insulin resistance are associated with inflammation.

Risk of Type 2 Diabetes: Persistent sleep deprivation is associated with an increased risk of developing type 2 diabetes. Prioritizing adequate sleep is a proactive measure for diabetes prevention.

Blood Pressure Regulation:
Quality sleep contributes to the regulation of blood pressure, and hypertension is linked to impaired glucose metabolism. Controlling blood pressure is essential for overall cardiovascular health and blood sugar control.

Overall Metabolic Health:
A consistent sleep routine supports overall metabolic health, influencing factors such as lipid metabolism, appetite regulation, and hormonal balance—essential components for maintaining blood sugar levels.

For those focused on a blood sugar solution, incorporating good sleep hygiene practices, such as maintaining a regular sleep schedule, creating a comfortable sleep environment, and managing stress, is crucial. Prioritizing sufficient and quality sleep can significantly contribute to better blood sugar control and overall health.

CHAPTER SEVEN

Monitoring and Managing Blood Sugar Levels

Monitoring and managing blood sugar levels are crucial for individuals with diabetes or those at risk of developing it. Here's an overview of the key aspects of monitoring and managing blood sugar levels:

Blood Glucose Monitoring: Use a glucose meter to routinely measure your blood sugar levels. The determination of monitoring frequency and timing should be done in cooperation with healthcare specialists as they can differ.

Target Blood Sugar Ranges:
Set and understand target blood sugar ranges with the guidance of healthcare providers. This helps in determining whether blood sugar levels are within the desired parameters.

Medication Management:
For individuals with diabetes, taking prescribed
medications (insulin or oral medications) as
directed by healthcare providers is crucial.
Adherence to medication regimens helps
control blood sugar levels.

Healthy Eating:
Follow a balanced diet with controlled
carbohydrate intake. Spread meals throughout
the day to avoid large spikes in blood sugar
levels. Consult with a registered dietitian for
personalized meal planning.

Regular Physical Activity:
Engage in regular exercise as it helps improve
insulin sensitivity and supports blood sugar
control. Develop an exercise routine tailored to
individual capabilities and preferences.

Weight Management:
Achieve and maintain a healthy weight. Losing
excess weight, if applicable, can improve
insulin sensitivity and overall blood sugar
regulation.

Stress management: Engage in
stress-relieving activities like yoga, deep
breathing, or meditation. Managing stress is
crucial since long-term stress can affect blood
sugar levels.

Regular Medical Check-ups:
Schedule regular check-ups with healthcare
professionals. Monitor blood pressure,
cholesterol levels, and kidney function, as
these can influence blood sugar control.

- Educate oneself about diabetes management
and self-care practices. This includes
understanding how different foods, activities,
and lifestyle factors affect blood sugar levels.

Record Keeping:
- Keep a log or use digital tools to record blood sugar levels, meals, medications, and activities. This information helps identify patterns and allows healthcare providers to make informed adjustments.

Emergency Preparedness:
- Know how to respond to low or high blood sugar levels. Carry necessary supplies, such as glucose tablets or insulin, and educate family members or caregivers on emergency procedures.

Self-Monitoring Techniques

 Self-monitoring techniques are essential for individuals focused on a blood sugar solution, particularly those managing diabetes. Here are key self-monitoring techniques:

Glucose Monitoring:
Use a glucose meter to regularly check blood sugar levels. Follow the recommended testing frequency as advised by healthcare professionals.

Continuous Glucose Monitoring (CGM):
Consider using CGM systems for real-time monitoring. CGM devices provide continuous updates on glucose levels, trends, and alerts for potential highs or lows.

Blood Sugar Log:
Keep a detailed blood sugar log to track readings, meals, physical activity, and medications. This log helps identify patterns and provides valuable information for healthcare providers.

Target Blood Sugar Ranges:
Understand and set target blood sugar ranges in collaboration with healthcare professionals. Aim to keep blood sugar levels within these specified parameters.

Meal Planning:
Learn to estimate and manage carbohydrate intake. Use tools like food diaries or mobile apps to track meals and their impact on blood sugar levels.

Exercise Monitoring:
Monitor the effects of physical activity on blood
sugar levels. Keep track of the type, duration,
and intensity of exercises to understand their
impact.

Medication Adherence:
Adhere to prescribed medication regimens.
Use medication reminders or pill organizers to
ensure consistency in taking medications as
directed by healthcare providers.

Symptom Recognition:
Be aware of symptoms associated with both
high and low blood sugar levels. Promptly
address any unusual symptoms and seek
medical advice if needed.

Regular Health Check-ups:
Schedule routine check-ups with healthcare
professionals to assess overall health,
including blood pressure, cholesterol levels,
and kidney function.

Hydration Monitoring:
- Monitor fluid intake, as dehydration can affect
blood sugar levels. Ensure adequate hydration,
especially during physical activity or in hot
weather.

Stress Management Techniques:
- Practice stress-reducing techniques such as
meditation, deep breathing, or relaxation
exercises. Monitor stress levels and their
potential impact on blood sugar.

Checks for Foot and Skin: - Frequently
examine your feet and skin for any indications
of anomalies, infections, or ulcers. Inform
medical professionals of any concerns as soon
as possible.

Weight Tracking:
- Maintain a healthy weight through regular monitoring. Track weight changes and discuss them with healthcare providers to make necessary adjustments to the management plan.

Sleep Patterns:
- Monitor sleep patterns and address any issues affecting sleep quality. Aim for consistent sleep routines to support overall well-being and blood sugar control.

Effective self-monitoring requires education, awareness, and consistency. It empowers individuals to actively participate in their blood sugar management, make informed decisions, and collaborate effectively with healthcare professionals for optimal outcomes.

Medication Management and Senior Health

Medication Adherence:
Seniors should strictly adhere to their prescribed medication regimen, taking medications at the recommended times and in the correct doses. Skipping doses or altering medication schedules can impact blood sugar control.

Regular Medication Review:
Schedule regular medication reviews with healthcare professionals. As seniors may take multiple medications for various health conditions, it's important to ensure there are no interactions that could affect blood sugar levels.

Blood Sugar Monitoring:
Consistently monitor blood sugar levels to
assess the effectiveness of medications.
Regular monitoring helps determine whether
adjustments are needed in the type or dosage
of medications.

Insulin Administration:
If insulin is part of the treatment plan, seniors
should be trained on proper insulin
administration techniques. This includes
understanding insulin types, injection sites, and
storage.

Side Effect Awareness:
Seniors should be aware of potential side
effects associated with their diabetes
medications. Any unusual symptoms or
reactions should be reported to healthcare
providers promptly.

Collaboration with Healthcare Providers:
Maintain open communication with healthcare professionals. Discuss any concerns, changes in health status, or challenges with medication adherence to receive timely guidance and adjustments.

Medication Storage:
Properly store medications according to their specific requirements. Ensure medications are kept in a cool, dry place, away from direct sunlight, and out of reach of children.

Emergency Preparedness:
Seniors should be educated on what to do in case of missed doses, emergencies, or changes in health status. Emergency contact information and a list of medications should be easily accessible.

Comprehensive Health Management:
Address overall health concerns that may
impact diabetes management. This includes
managing conditions such as hypertension,
high cholesterol, or kidney issues that can
influence blood sugar levels.

Geriatric Assessment:
- Consider a geriatric assessment to evaluate
the overall health and well-being of seniors.
This can help tailor a comprehensive
healthcare plan that considers the unique
needs of older individuals.

Nutrition and Medication Interaction:
- Seniors should be mindful of how their
medications may interact with their diet. For
example, some medications may require
adjustments based on meal timing or nutrient
intake.

Regular Check-ups:
- Schedule regular check-ups with healthcare providers to monitor diabetes management and assess the impact of medications on overall health.

Medication management for seniors with diabetes is a collaborative effort between healthcare professionals, seniors, and caregivers. It involves ongoing education, monitoring, and adjustments to ensure an effective blood sugar solution while considering the specific needs and challenges associated with senior health.

CHAPTER EIGHT

Social Support and Community Engagement

Social support and community engagement play vital roles in achieving and maintaining a blood sugar solution, especially for individuals managing diabetes. Here's how they contribute:

Emotional Support:

Social connections provide emotional support, which is crucial for managing the psychological aspects of living with diabetes. A supportive network can help individuals cope with stress, anxiety, and the challenges associated with blood sugar management.

Shared Experiences:
Engaging with others who have similar experiences fosters a sense of understanding and empathy. Sharing strategies, successes, and challenges creates a supportive community that can enhance motivation and confidence.

Encouragement for Healthy Behaviors:
Social support encourages the adoption of healthy behaviors. Whether it's engaging in regular exercise, following a balanced diet, or adhering to medication regimens, having a supportive network reinforces positive habits.

Peer Accountability:
Community engagement provides a level of accountability. Knowing that others share similar health goals encourages individuals to stay committed to their blood sugar solution plans.

Education and Information Sharing:
Social groups and communities are valuable sources of information and education. Participants can share insights, resources, and updates on the latest advancements in blood sugar management.

Practical Tips and Advice:
Interacting with others facing similar challenges allows for the exchange of practical tips and advice. Learning from real-life experiences can be invaluable in refining one's approach to blood sugar control.

Lifestyle Integration:
Community engagement promotes the integration of a blood sugar solution into daily life. By participating in group activities and discussions, individuals can discover practical ways to manage their condition within the context of their social and cultural environments.

Supportive Family and Friends:
The involvement of family and friends in a person's blood sugar solution can have a significant impact. Educating loved ones about diabetes, its management, and the importance of a healthy lifestyle creates a supportive environment at home.

Community Programs and Workshops:
Attend community programs, workshops, or support groups specifically focused on diabetes management. These can offer structured education, expert advice, and opportunities to connect with others on a similar health journey.

Diminished Sensations of Isolation:
Diabetes can occasionally exacerbate isolated sensations. By fostering a feeling of connection and belonging, social support and community involvement work to counteract this and lessen the emotional toll that the illness takes.

Online Communities and Forums:
- Participate in online forums or social media groups dedicated to diabetes management. These platforms offer a virtual space for information sharing, support, and connection with a diverse range of individuals.

Community Events:
- Attend local health fairs, events, or wellness programs. These activities often provide opportunities to learn, engage with healthcare professionals, and connect with others interested in blood sugar management.

Incorporating social support and community engagement into a blood sugar solution not only enhances motivation but also creates a collaborative and enriching environment that contributes to long-term success in managing diabetes.

Building a Supportive Network

Building a supportive network is essential for individuals working towards a blood sugar solution, particularly those managing diabetes. Here's how to establish and strengthen a supportive network:

Family and Friends:
Educate and involve family and friends in your blood sugar solution. Share information about your condition, treatment plan, and lifestyle changes. Seek their understanding and support in maintaining a healthy environment.

Diabetes Support Groups:
Join local or online diabetes support groups where individuals facing similar challenges share experiences, advice, and encouragement. These groups provide a sense of community and understanding.

Healthcare Professionals:
Establish open communication with healthcare
providers. Discuss your goals, challenges, and
concerns related to blood sugar management.
Regularly update them on your progress and
seek guidance on adjustments to your plan.

Nutritionist or Dietitian:
Consult with a nutritionist or dietitian to create
a personalized meal plan. Involve them in your
blood sugar solution journey, and regularly
discuss any adjustments needed based on
your preferences and health goals.

Exercise Partners: Look for a training partner
or enroll in group fitness programs. Having a
companion can increase the enjoyment of
physical activity and foster mutual incentive to
continue exercising, both of which are critical
for blood sugar regulation.

Mentorship:
Seek guidance from someone who has
successfully managed their blood sugar levels.
A mentor can share practical tips, offer
insights, and provide emotional support based
on their own experiences.

Workplace Support:
Inform colleagues and supervisors about your
condition, especially if it may impact your work
schedule or require accommodations. A
supportive work environment can contribute to
stress reduction and better blood sugar
management.

Online Communities:
Explore online forums, social media groups, or
health apps focused on blood sugar
management. Engaging with individuals
virtually allows for continuous support and
information sharing.

Educational Classes:
Attend diabetes education classes or workshops. These settings offer opportunities to connect with others while gaining valuable knowledge about managing blood sugar levels.

Regular Check-ins:
- Schedule regular check-ins with members of your support network. Share updates on your progress, discuss challenges, and celebrate successes together. Consistent communication fosters a sense of accountability and encouragement.

Wellness Programs:
- Participate in wellness programs offered by local community centers or healthcare organizations. These programs often cover a variety of health-related topics, providing a supportive environment for holistic well-being.

Communication Skills:
- Develop effective communication skills to express your needs, concerns, and boundaries to your support network. Clear communication helps in establishing expectations and fostering understanding.

Building a supportive network involves proactive communication, education, and shared experiences. It creates an environment where individuals feel empowered, encouraged, and understood in their journey towards achieving and maintaining optimal blood sugar levels.

Community Resources for Senior Health

Community resources for senior health play a crucial role in providing support, services, and opportunities for older individuals to maintain and enhance their well-being. Here are common community resources for senior health:

1. **Senior Centers:**
These centers offer a variety of activities, including social events, fitness classes, educational programs, and health screenings. They provide a space for seniors to connect, engage, and stay active.

2. **Nutrition Programs:**
Community-based nutrition programs, such as Meals on Wheels, deliver nutritious meals to homebound seniors. Some centers also offer congregate meal programs where seniors can share a meal in a communal setting.

3. Exercise Classes and Fitness Programs: Local community centers often organize exercise classes tailored to seniors, promoting physical activity and overall health. This may include activities like yoga, tai chi, or water aerobics.

4. **Transportation Services:**
Transportation programs assist seniors in getting to medical appointments, grocery shopping, and social activities. Accessible transportation services are particularly beneficial for those with mobility challenges.

5. **Health Screenings and Clinics:**

Community health fairs and clinics provide access to preventive health services, screenings, and vaccinations. These events often focus on addressing specific health concerns relevant to seniors.

6. **Support Groups:**

Support groups for seniors dealing with health conditions, caregiving responsibilities, or specific life changes offer emotional support and a sense of community. These groups may be organized by community centers, healthcare organizations, or local churches.

7. **Educational Workshops:**

Workshops on topics like managing chronic conditions, understanding medications, and navigating healthcare systems help seniors stay informed and empowered in making health-related decisions.

8. **Home Health Services:**
Home health agencies offer services such as home healthcare, home safety assessments, and assistance with activities of daily living. These resources support seniors in maintaining independence while addressing their health needs.

9. **Elder Abuse Prevention Programs:**
Community resources focused on elder abuse prevention raise awareness and provide support for seniors facing abuse or exploitation. These programs often include educational initiatives and confidential reporting mechanisms.

10. **Volunteer Opportunities:**
- Volunteer programs provide seniors with opportunities to contribute to their communities. This can have positive effects on mental health and foster a sense of purpose and social connection.

11. **Legal Aid Services:**

- Legal aid services catered to seniors can assist with issues like estate planning, advance directives, and accessing public benefits. These services help seniors navigate legal matters related to their well-being.

12. **Recreation and Leisure Activities:**

- Community resources for recreation and leisure activities, such as senior clubs, hobby groups, or cultural organizations, offer opportunities for seniors to engage in activities they enjoy and maintain a sense of fulfillment.

13. **Aging and Disability Resource Centers (ADRCs):**

- ADRCs provide information and assistance on a range of services for seniors and individuals with disabilities. They serve as centralized points for accessing support, guidance, and resources.

14. **Social Services Agencies:**

- Local social services agencies offer a variety of assistance programs, including financial support, housing assistance, and counseling services, to address the comprehensive needs of seniors.

Accessing and utilizing these community resources can significantly contribute to the overall well-being of seniors, supporting their health, independence, and quality of life.

Addressing Common Concerns about Blood Sugar in Seniors

Addressing common concerns about blood sugar in seniors is essential for their overall health and well-being. Here are some common concerns and ways to address them:

1. **Hypoglycemia (Low Blood Sugar):**
Concern: Seniors may experience episodes of low blood sugar, leading to symptoms like confusion, weakness, or dizziness.
Address: Encourage regular, balanced meals, and snacks. Adjust medication doses if needed. Ensure seniors have a source of fast-acting glucose, like glucose tablets, to raise blood sugar in case of an emergency.

2. Hyperglycemia (High Blood Sugar):

Concern: Consistently high blood sugar levels can lead to complications, including increased risk of cardiovascular disease and nerve damage.

Address: Monitor blood sugar levels regularly. Adjust diet and medication plans as advised by healthcare professionals. Encourage physical activity to improve insulin sensitivity.

3. Medication Management:

Concern: Seniors may face challenges in managing medications, including confusion about doses or forgetting to take them.

Address: Simplify medication regimens whenever possible. Use pill organizers or medication reminders. Regularly review medications with healthcare providers to ensure appropriateness and minimal side effects.

4. Cognitive Decline:

Concern: Cognitive decline may impact a senior's ability to manage their blood sugar effectively.

Address: Involve family members or caregivers in the management plan. Simplify instructions and use visual aids. Regularly reassess the individual's ability to self-manage, considering their cognitive health.

5. Limited Physical Activity:

Concern: Reduced mobility or limitations in physical activity can contribute to blood sugar control challenges.

Address: Encourage low-impact exercises, such as walking or chair exercises. Consider activities that align with the individual's abilities and preferences. Consult with healthcare providers for safe exercise recommendations.

6. **Diet Challenges:**
Concern: Dietary issues, such as difficulty chewing or lack of appetite, can impact nutrition and blood sugar control.
Address: Modify textures of food if needed. Offer small, nutrient-dense meals. Work with a dietitian to create a personalized meal plan that accommodates dietary restrictions and preferences.

7. **Dehydration:**
Concern: Seniors may be at risk of dehydration, which can affect blood sugar concentration.
Address: Encourage adequate fluid intake. Include hydrating foods like fruits and vegetables in the diet. Monitor for signs of dehydration, especially during hot weather or illnesses.

8. **Social Isolation:**

Concern: Seniors may face social isolation, impacting their mental well-being and potentially their ability to manage blood sugar.
Address: Foster social connections through community programs, support groups, or family involvement. Ensure regular check-ins and companionship to reduce feelings of isolation.

9. **Financial Constraints**:

Concern: Limited financial resources may affect access to healthy food options and medications.
Address: Connect seniors with community resources, such as nutrition assistance programs or prescription assistance programs. Explore cost-effective ways to maintain a healthy lifestyle.

10. **Regular Health Check-ups:**
- **Concern**: Seniors may neglect regular health check-ups, missing opportunities for preventive care and blood sugar monitoring.
- **Address**: Emphasize the importance of regular check-ups. Assist in scheduling appointments and accompany seniors to medical visits when needed.

Addressing these concerns requires a comprehensive and individualized approach. Collaborate with healthcare professionals, involve family members or caregivers, and tailor interventions to meet the unique needs of each senior. Regular communication and adjustments to the management plan are crucial for sustained blood sugar control.

CONCLUSION

In conclusion, implementing a blood sugar diet solution tailored for seniors involves a multifaceted approach that addresses their unique needs and challenges. The emphasis should be on promoting a balanced and nutrient-rich diet, incorporating delicious yet blood sugar-friendly recipes. Sample meal plans, rich in fiber, lean proteins, and healthy fats, can serve as valuable guides to support optimal blood sugar control.

Furthermore, recognizing the importance of lifestyle modifications is pivotal. Regular physical activity, stress management techniques, and sufficient sleep contribute significantly to improved blood sugar levels. Seniors can enhance their overall well-being by embracing these lifestyle changes, fostering a holistic approach to health.

Monitoring and managing blood sugar levels play a central role in the success of any blood sugar diet solution. Utilizing self-monitoring techniques, such as glucose monitoring, keeping detailed logs, and understanding target blood sugar ranges, empowers seniors to actively participate in their health journey. Regular communication with healthcare professionals ensures personalized guidance and timely adjustments to the management plan.

The significance of social support and community engagement cannot be overstated. Building a supportive network, both within the family and through community resources, creates an environment that encourages adherence to the blood sugar solution. Emotional support, shared experiences, and access to community programs contribute to the success of seniors in managing their blood sugar effectively.

Addressing common concerns related to blood sugar in seniors, from hypoglycemia to limited physical activity, requires careful consideration and individualized strategies. Recognizing the impact of cognitive decline, medication management challenges, and lifestyle limitations ensures a comprehensive and tailored approach to promoting health and preventing complications.

In navigating the complexities of blood sugar management for seniors, the integration of community resources becomes paramount. Senior centers, nutrition programs, exercise classes, and various support services play pivotal roles in providing the necessary assistance and opportunities for seniors to thrive in their pursuit of optimal blood sugar levels.

Ultimately, achieving a successful blood sugar diet solution for seniors necessitates a collaborative effort. Seniors, along with their healthcare professionals, family members, and community, can work together to create a supportive environment that prioritizes health, well-being, and a vibrant and fulfilling lifestyle in the golden years.

Thank you for taking the time to explore the intricacies of the Blood Sugar Diet Solution for Seniors. Your commitment to understanding the unique challenges and holistic strategies involved in managing blood sugar levels for older individuals is truly commendable. By investing in this knowledge, you contribute not only to the well-being of seniors but also to a healthier and more informed community. Your dedication to promoting a proactive and supportive approach to senior health is invaluable. Together, we can make a meaningful impact on the lives of our seniors, fostering vitality, and enhancing their quality of life. Thank you for being an advocate for health and wellness in our aging population.

Appendix

Glossary Of Terms Related To The Blood Sugar Diet Solution For Seniors

S/N	DESCRIPTION	FUNCTION
1	Blood Sugar Levels	The concentration of glucose in the bloodstream, measured in milligrams per deciliter (mg/dL) or millimoles per liter (mmol/L). Maintaining balanced blood sugar levels are crucial for overall health.

2	Insulin	a pancreatic hormone that aids in the uptake of glucose by cells, hence assisting in blood sugar regulation. Diabetes is characterized by either inadequate insulin production or the body's development of resistance to its effects.
3	Glucose Monitoring	The process of regularly checking blood sugar levels using a glucose meter to assess and manage diabetes.
4	Hypoglycemia	A condition characterized by abnormally

		low blood sugar levels, leading to symptoms like dizziness, confusion, and weakness.
5	Hyperglycemia	Elevated levels of blood sugar, often associated with diabetes, which can lead to complications if not managed effectively.
6	Carbohydrates	nutrients that, during digestion, are converted into glucose and are present in meals like grains, fruits, and vegetables. Controlling

		one's carbohydrate consumption is essential for controlling blood sugar.
7	A1c (Glycated Hemoglobin)	a blood test used to determine the blood sugar average during the previous two to three months. It is a crucial sign of long-term blood sugar regulation.
8	Dietary Fiber	Plant-based nutrients that are not fully digested, helping regulate blood sugar levels by slowing down the absorption of glucose.

9	Glycemic Index (GI)	A scale that assesses how rapidly carbs in diets boost blood sugar levels. Choosing foods with a lower GI can aid with blood sugar stabilization.
10	Insulin Resistance	A condition where cells do not respond effectively to insulin, leading to elevated blood sugar levels. It is a key factor in type 2 diabetes.
11	Ketones	substances created when fat is broken down by the body to provide

		energy. Uncontrolled diabetes can cause elevated ketone levels, which can result in diabetic ketoacidosis.
12	Metabolism	the method by which the body produces energy from food. For blood sugar control, metabolism must be understood and optimized.
13	Portion Control	Managing the size of food portions to regulate calorie intake and support healthy blood sugar levels.

14	Hydration	Maintaining adequate fluid intake, as dehydration can impact blood sugar concentration.
15	Community Resources	Services and programs within the community that support seniors in achieving a blood sugar diet solution, including nutrition programs, exercise classes, and support groups.
16	Cognitive Decline	A reduction in cognitive abilities, such as memory and problem-solving skills, which can

		impact a senior's ability to manage their blood sugar effectively.
17	Medication Adherence	Consistently following prescribed medication regimens to control blood sugar levels and manage diabetes.